This Is Me

(And You)

Warren Knowlton

ISBN 978-1-0980-7929-1 (paperback)
ISBN 978-1-0980-7930-7 (digital)

Christian Faith Publishing, Inc.
832 Park Avenue
Meadville, PA 16335
www.christianfaithpublishing.com

Printed in the United States of America

Values and Principles

Exploring your
values and principles
can help you live the
life you want.
Start a list of your
own of
sayings or
thoughts
that express who you are
or want to be.
Add to it as you discover
words
from books or media
or that you
formulate.
Make several copies
and post them
where you will see them
and continually
be reminded
of
them.

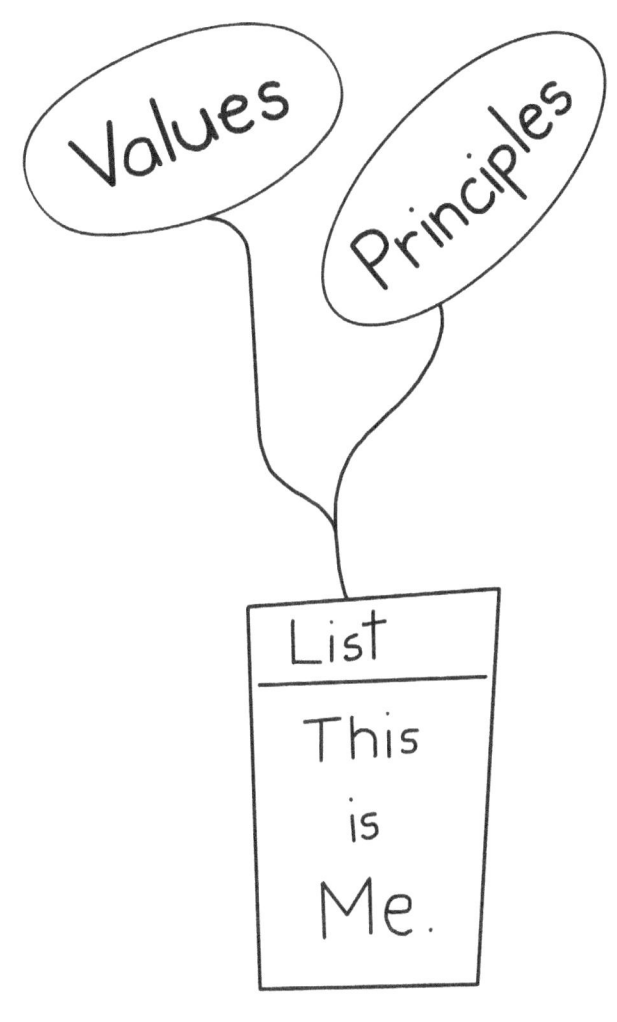

Bliss

(A state or feeling of perfect happiness)

Bliss
is
letting go of
yesterday.
Remembering a day
of joy.
Anticipating tomorrow
as a plan fulfilled.
Being in the now.
Seeing beauty in the
ordinary.
Sharing and being
with love.
Accepting what
is.

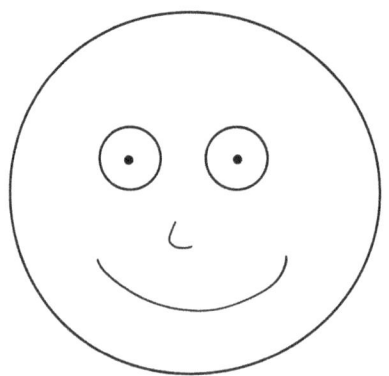

Find and Press
Trigger Points Daily

When a stretch hurts,
back off just a little,
then hunt for trigger points
in the muscle moving away
from the pain.
To find trigger points
push on the muscle with
fingers, thumb, tool, ball, stick,
or foam roller.
Release pressure, move one-half inch,
repeat over and over as you move
along a muscle.
A spot that hurts when pushed on,
deserves about ten to fifteen
seconds of pressure.
Just enough to feel some pain.
You can also use isometric exercise
to ease trigger points.
Move into an easy stretch.
Tighten a muscle by pushing on something,
pulling on something,
or intentional tightening.
Hold for fifteen seconds,
then relax and flex the muscle.

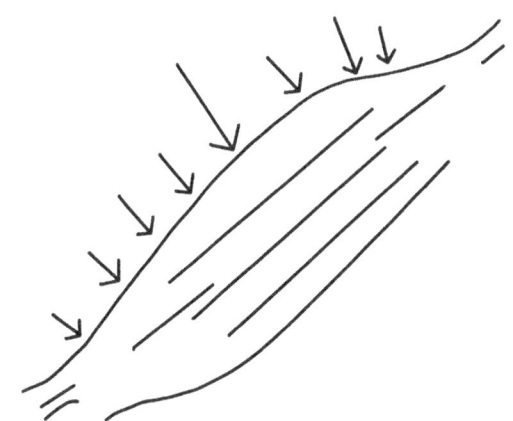

Stretch Daily

Stretching is Yoga Lite.
Move big muscles
in various ways
as far as they
want to go.
If you feel no pain
all is good.
If you feel pain
slow down.
Move judiciously
into the edge of
pain, and then
back away.
Do it over and over.
Sometimes muscles
need to rest to heal.
Respect that.
Don't bounce your stretch.
Ease into the full movement available,
hold a bit, then back out.
Move on to the next stretch.
Get a routine
you can do
daily.

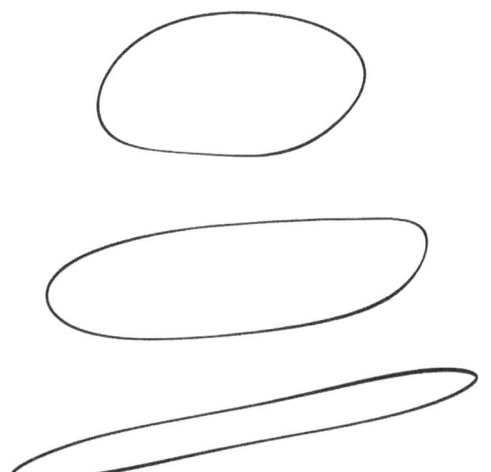

Be Kind, Do Good

Or be
nice and caring.
Some people think
they can be good
and not kind.
It's a choice.
I think all good
can be done with kindness. I think this summarizes
Religious teaching.
If you are not religious
it describes a
moral behavior.
Ask yourself,
Am I being kind?
Is this good for the
earth, people,
family, friends,
strangers?
Are you guided
by this when
working, playing, resting?
Is it so ingrained in you
that it is automatic?

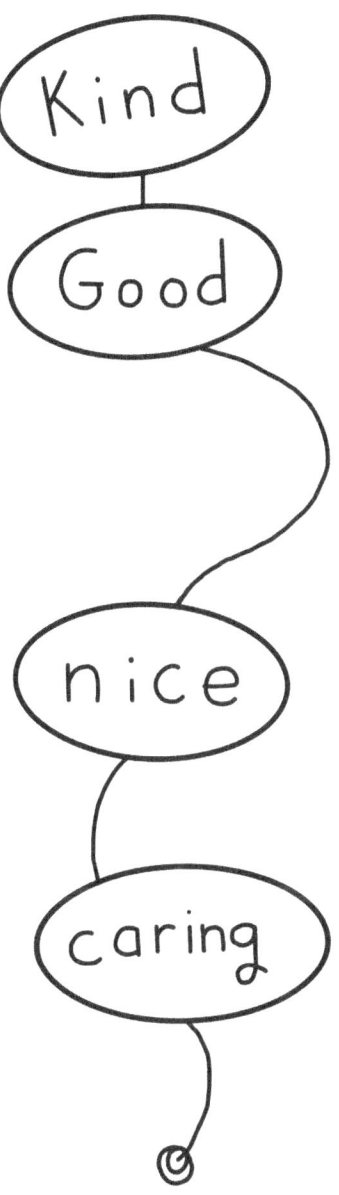

Look for the Good in Everybody

Sometimes it may be
hard to do.
That is when it is
most important
to do it.
This is a useful mindset
for dealing with anybody.
Those you love
deserve a daily dose
of being seen as good.
More is better.
Look for the good
in yourself.
How do you
put it to use?
Political parties.
Both sides have
good points.
Start there.

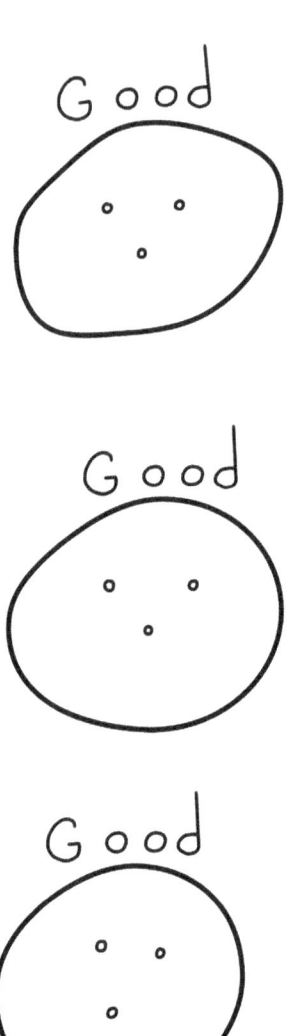

Do Something Worthwhile Every Day

Worthwhile is
whatever
I decide it is.
If I'm sick
and lying in bed,
then getting
up to pee
is worthwhile.
If I need to get
some work done,
getting it done
is worthwhile.
Practicing my music
is worthwhile.
Getting some exercise
is worthwhile.
Eating for health
is worthwhile.
Putting tools away
is worthwhile.
Saying
I Love You.

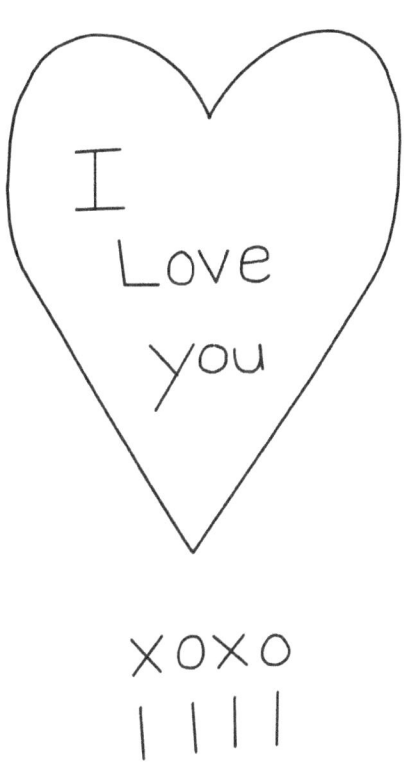

Keep Tweaking Until it Works

Most ideas need to be
Refined,
Tested,
Evaluated,
Redone.

Write a paper.
Read it,
Correct it,
Print it,
Let it sit
a while.
Revise.

Cleaning.
Sort,
Make piles,
Throw away,
Give away,
Put away,
Start over.

Making a list.
Cross out what you did.
See what you are not
going to do.
Make a new list.

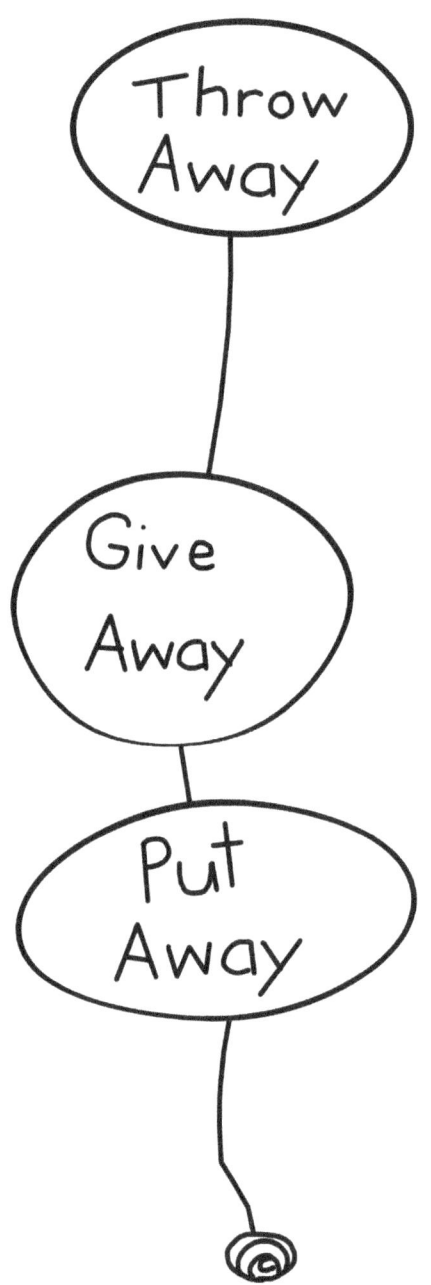

Pride

Having a goal.
Working toward it.
Achieving, step by step
Growth.
Sharing your achievements.
Teaching what you know to
Others.
Satisfied that you
are doing
Good
for mankind.
Ready to take on new
challenges,
interests,
and learning as you go.
Sometimes wrong,
willing to change to be
Better.
Thanking those
who helped you
along the
way.

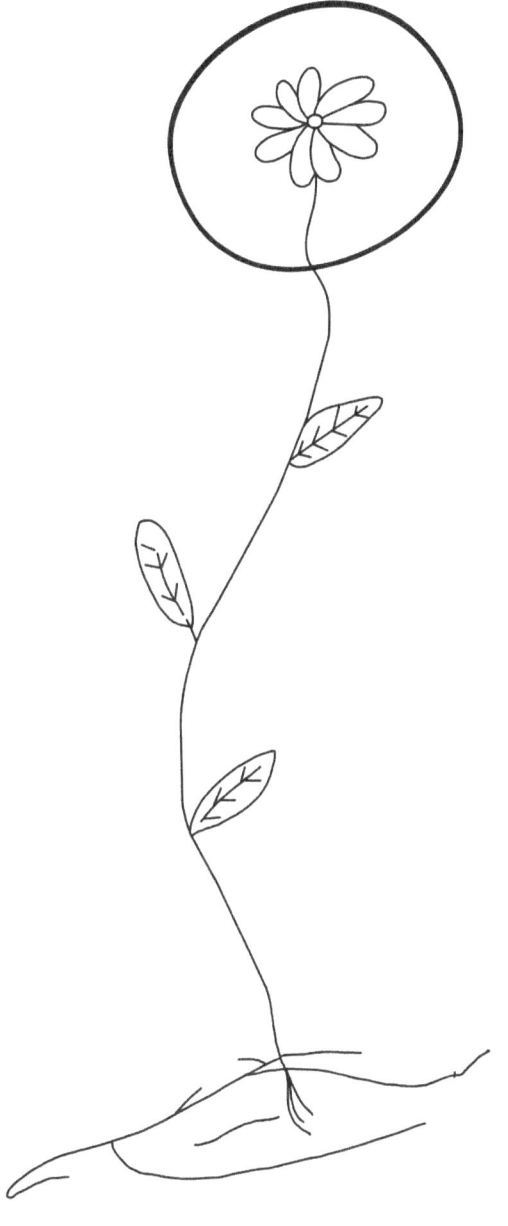

Take a deep breath and relax.
Breathe from the diaphragm.

Move your stomach out.
Move upward toward your shoulder.
Move both together.
Hold for five seconds.
Exhale.
Whenever you feel stress,
take several deep slow breaths.
Think "relax" to yourself
as you exhale.
When at a stoplight waiting,
count down from ten.
Breathe deeply.
Flex your fingers
to release tension.
Find time each day to
turn everything off.
Sitting in the quiet,
relax muscles,
breathe deeply.

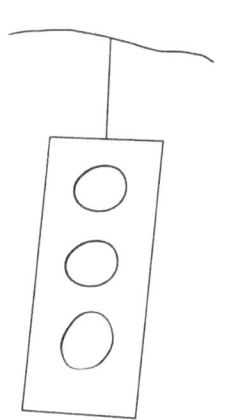

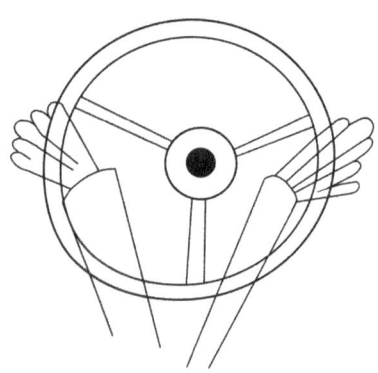

Move toward Contentment

(Satisfaction)

If you wish you could do something,
start to prepare and act on it.
Then accept the results.
Then daily work on it.
Make a list and then cross off
items as you do them.

GRATITUDE
Think of things to be thankful for.
Thank people often.
What do you see around you
that you appreciate?
Open doors for others
and let somebody
go ahead of you.

MEDITATE
Turn everything off.
Breathe deeply.
Let thoughts come and
then let go of
them.

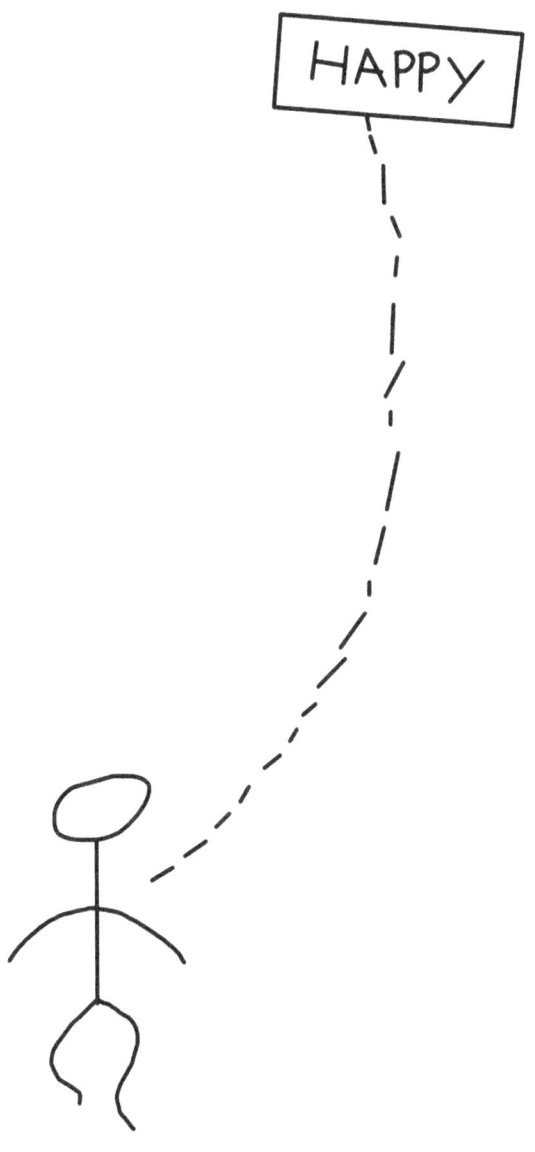

Guilt and Anger
are useless feelings.

They can be real feelings.
You feel guilt.
Do something to relieve it.
Say "I am sorry."
Talk to an empty chair as if it
is the person.
Then switch parts.
Resolve it and move on.
What can you do with anger?
Hurt somebody? Not a good idea.
Yell. Not if it raises your
blood pressure.
Count to ten. Take a few deep breaths.
Walk away. Stop and start over.
So calm down. What can you
do to resolve the feeling?
Do it. Then stop the behavior
leading to the feeling.
Replace with Forgiveness.

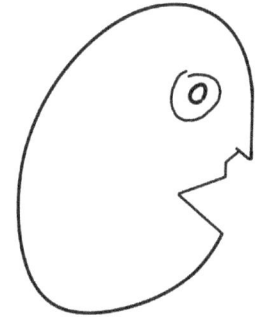
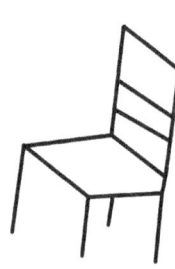

No Pride, No Shame
I Am What I Am

When performing in front of people
it helps to let go of
thoughts
about them or you.
Just do what you do.
Mistakes are
opportunities
to change direction,
or to simply keep going.
Notice what can be improved.
Practice with the aim
to correct mistakes.
Practice like it matters.
Perform like it doesn't.
When it comes to
other people,
you don't know what other people
are thinking.
It probably is not about
you.

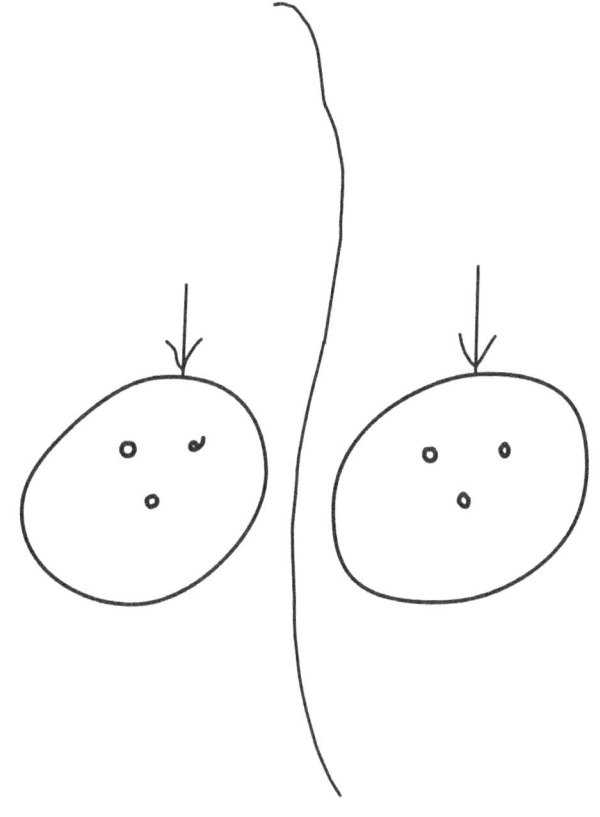

Be in the Here and Now
Observe

When you think
or worry about something
that happened in the past,
stop.
It's over.
Planning for the future
can be useful,
but repeating the same thought
over and over
isn't.
Put your plan into
action.
Look around and notice
what is there.
When you are listening to somebody,
do so with your
full attention.
Right now, right here,
is generally a safe place.
Take it in.

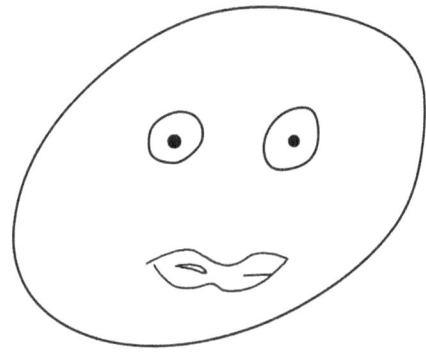

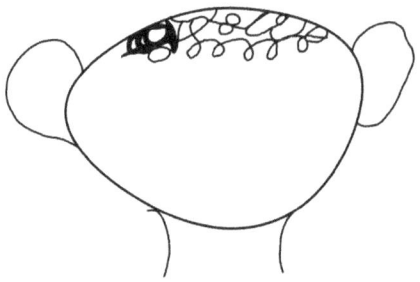

Values and Principles

Joys and Pleasures

It's No Big Deal

In the long run it isn't.
So it doesn't need to be so
in the short run.
No matter what happens
it needs a calm,
thoughtful approach
to resolve it.
Don't yell.
Don't argue.
Now focus on
what can be done to
make things better.
Allow yourself to breathe and relax.
If you need "toys" that
are a big deal
maybe you can
make some
adjustment.
Don't let situations
turn into a
big deal.
Choose your behavior.

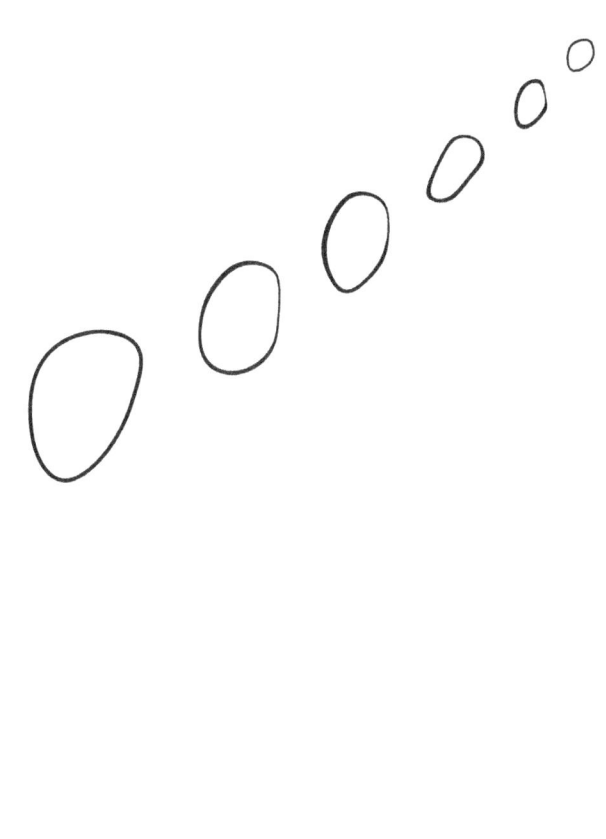

I'll Do One More --------

This is a trick
I learned driving tractor
in a field.
Want to stop.
Do one more round.
And then do one
more.
Don't
do this when eating.
cleaning—yes,
drinking—no,
saying thank you—yes.
Use common sense
to decide when
to use this
and when to
not.

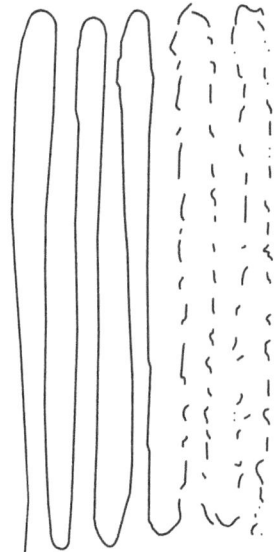

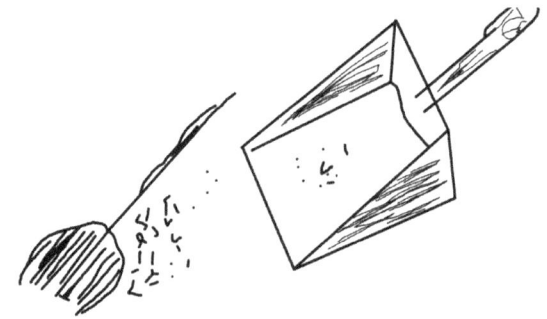

Postpone and Substitute

(diet)

The urge to eat something
will often weaken,
or even die out,
if given some time
and a distraction.
Give yourself five to ten minutes.
Then look for something
better to eat.
What if you feel
anger building up?
Allow some time
to deep breathe
and relax.
Think of a way
to be caring.
Feel like a nap?
Go for a
five-minute walk
outside.

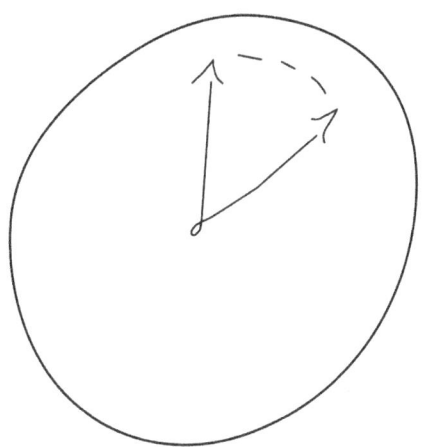

A Diet Starts in the Grocery Store. Don't Bring it Home.

Make a grocery list.
Include food that is good for you.
Avoid sugar and white flour
as ingredients.
Include fruits
and vegetables.
Choose meat carefully.
Eggs are okay.
Eat a green leafy salad daily.

Buy only what you will eat
to cut down on waste.

Be healthy by eating food good for you.

Don't forget to get some exercise.

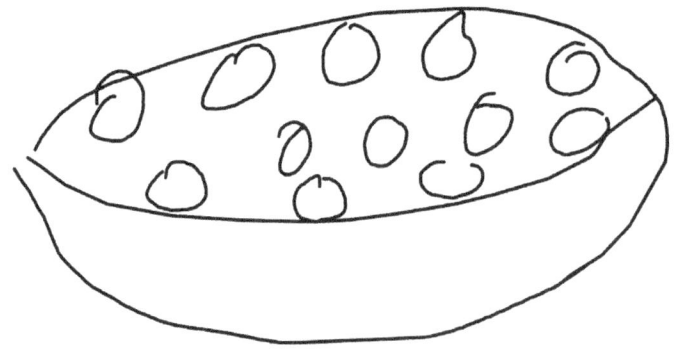

Metabolism

The process by which food is used for tissue growth or energy production.

If you want more energy
or help losing weight,
what can you do to
up your metabolism?
Try these ideas.

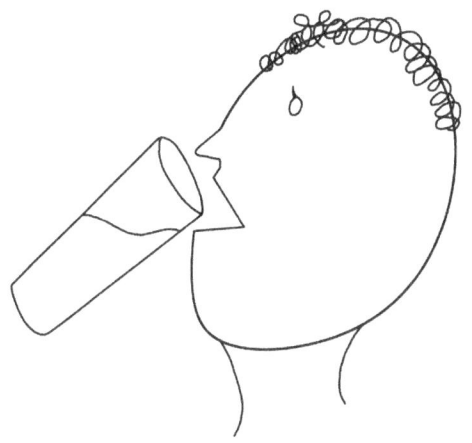

Drink a couple of glasses
of water in the morning.
Wait an hour before eating.
Hopefully you will burn
fat for energy.
Then break your fast—breakfast.

After you are done eating,
get another boost by
exercising large muscles
full blast for five minutes.
Running in place, Push-ups,
Sit-ups, Leg lifts, Touching your toes.

Moderation in All of Life

Too much of something is
obsessive or compulsive.

Food—Use a small plate.

Exercise—Balance with rest and recovery.

Cleaning—Do enough to live with.

Travel—Remember to appreciate home.

Love—Dish it out often in small amounts.

Work—Pace yourself.

Play—Temper with work.

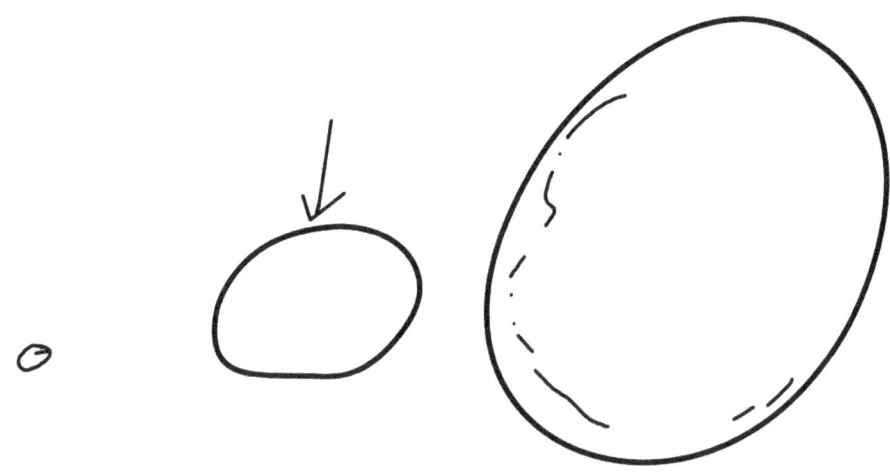

If It Bothers Me
It's My Job to Fix It Myself.

This is how the dishes get done.
The floor cleaned.
The laundry done.
The lawn mowed.
Don't expect somebody else
to be bothered as much as you
about your dirty socks.
If I don't want to,
or don't know how, I'll pay
somebody else to do it.
Some things don't bother me
that need to get done.
Choose to do things
that need doing.
Work with significant others
what chores you do
and they do.
Reward yourself if
needed to encourage
behavior.

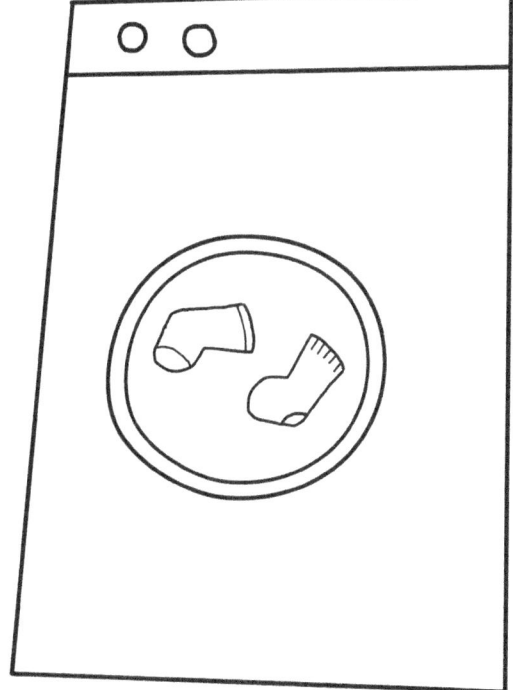

Make a List
Prioritize

I collect envelopes I get from the mail. I have a stack by a chair. When I need to write myself a note, I take one off the stack. Fold it into thirds, and it fits in a shirt pocket.

Before I go to town,
I make a list.
When I'm out of food,
I make a list.
When I'm not sure
what to do,
I make list.
When I learn to play a song,
I add it to a list.
When I'm learning a song,
I put it on a list.
When somebody on TV
is covering several points,
I make a list.
Sometimes I go through my lists
and throw away old ones
that have past their
time.

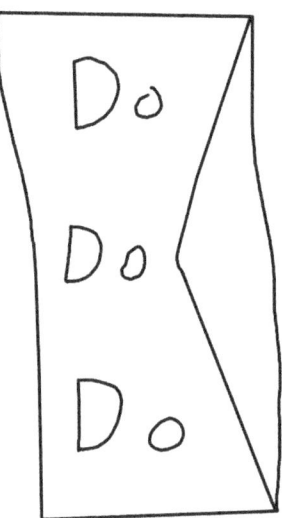

Wealth

Make more money
than you spend.
Save the rest.
This is how people
get rich.
Pay full amount on
credit cards monthly.
Define your needs.
Define your wants.
Budget for your needs.
Limit your wants.
Get the money
ahead of time
to pay for them.
Do things you enjoy
that cost little.
Have a hobby
that you enjoy
to spend time on.
Spend times with
people you
enjoy being with.

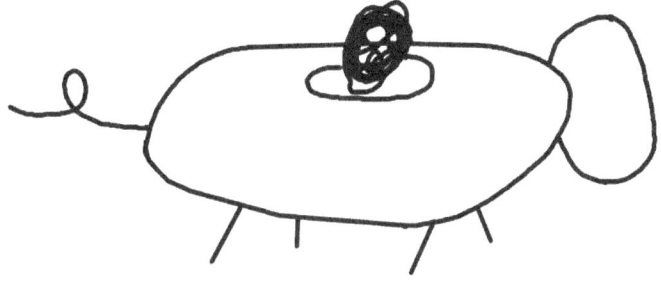

I Won't Let Somebody Else Determine How I Feel

I am responsible for my
feelings toward others.
I will not blame others
for how I feel.
I will own my choice not
to react to others.
If I am upset about a
situation and I am
responding to
somebody else,
LET IT GO.

Does *LOVE* fit this?

This is mostly about *NOT*
responding to negative
vibes.
Your *SELF-WORTH*
is your responsibility.
Others can be
tuned out
or, if rewarding,
accepted.

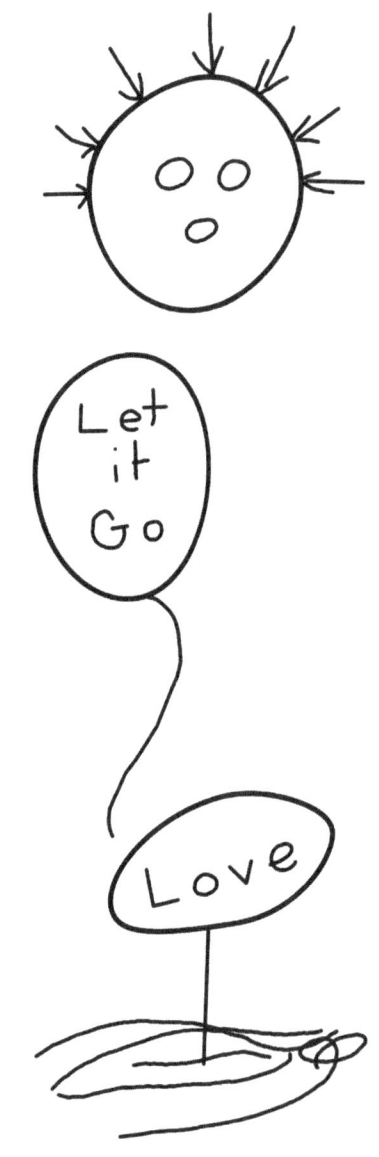

It Doesn't Matter to Me

What I do does matter.
I have no control
of others.
Detach from other's drama.
When I disagree with
somebody on how
to do something,
this is the time
to remember this.
It is helpful
to discover
what matters to others.
Maybe I can help
make it happen.
When somebody asks me
to do something I'm
not obliged.
Only if I am willing.
How others live their life
or what they believe
is not my concern.
It is when I think
it matters that
I get uptight.

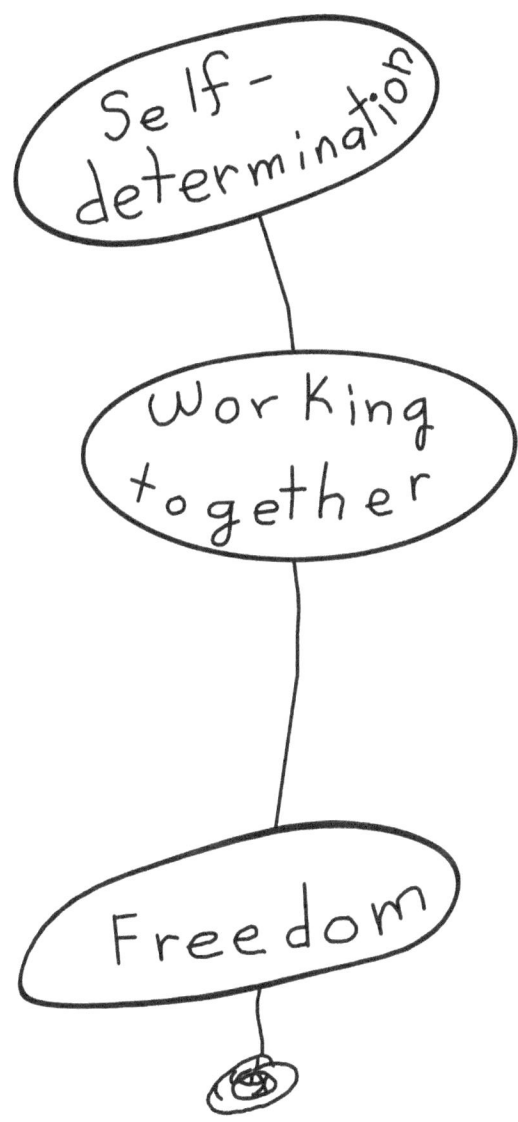

Use Your Strength
Work on Your Weakness

Do you know your strengths?
How can you use them?
List your strengths.
Choose how to use them.
Use all your strengths.
Decide which one you
want to
excel at.
Choose which weakness
you want to work on.
Spend some time daily
to get better.

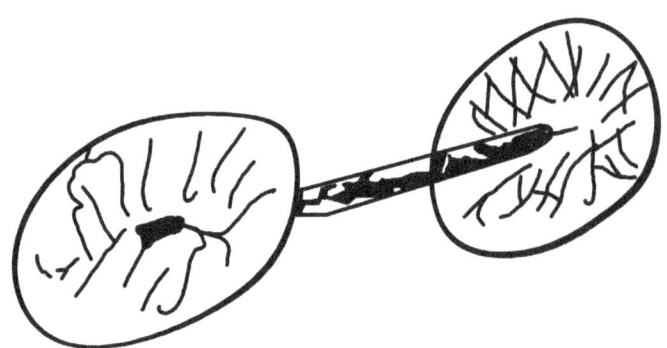

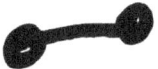

Big Stuff
Then Little Stuff

One time I cut down some trees in the yard.
I hooked on to the trunks with a chain and a tractor
then pulled them into a waste pasture.
It looked so much **better.**
Then I started to notice little branches.
I went around picking up branches.
Then I saw twigs.
I used a rake to rake up twigs.
Then I saw some holes that
needed filled.
The same process
happens
when learning to play
an instrument.
When cleaning a room.
When fixing my
mind.
Look for the
elephant
in the room.
Get it out.
Then clean up the
shit.

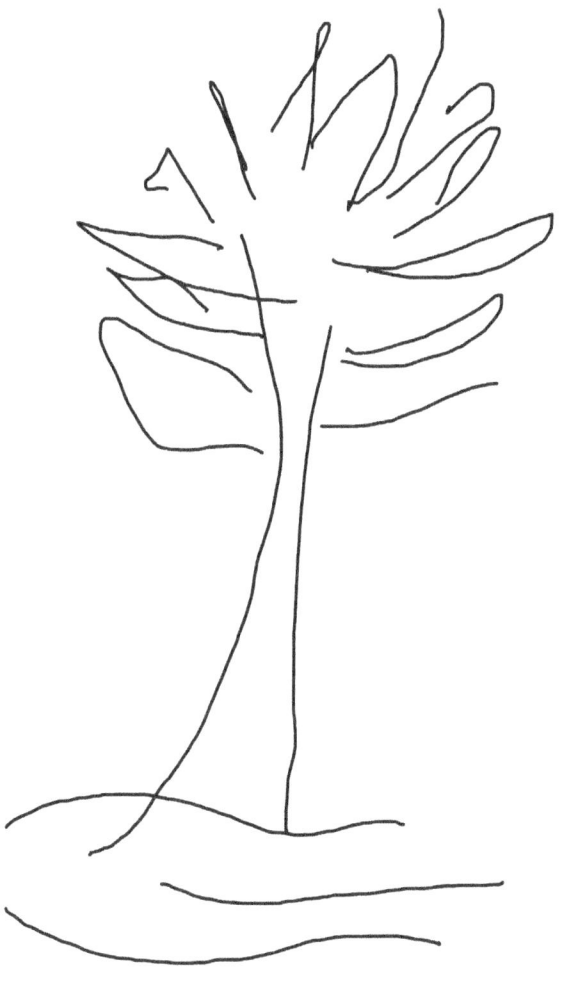

Dwell on Joys and Pleasures

Be intentional
about setting
aside time
to dwell on joys
and pleasures.
Make a list.
Smile.
Recognize
and appreciate
JOYS and
PLEASURES
as they
occur during the
day.
Create activities that you
enjoy.
Find pleasure
in regular
activities.
Eating
Talking
Reading
Watching TV
Resting.

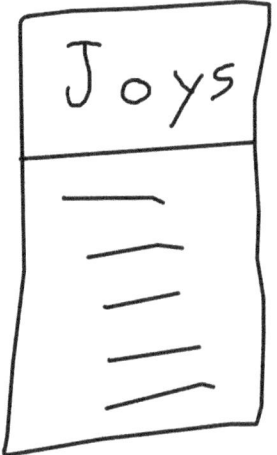

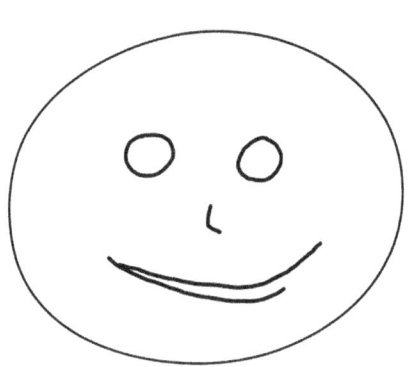

About the Author

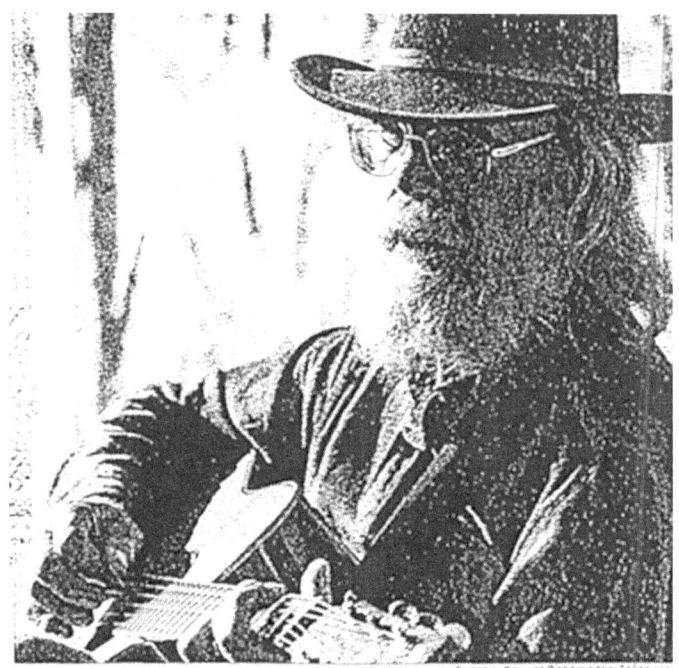

Guitar player Warren Knowlton with the Torrington Fiddlers open the morning with some soft and graceful playing as the dew disappears for the Pancake Breakfast in the park for the LaGrange Mini Festival.

Warren Knowlton, in college, studied to be an elementary teacher with music as a second teaching field. Then he got his master's degree in guidance and counseling. Then when his mother became ill, he came back to the family farm and spent forty years farming. During that time, he helped form the Torrington Fiddlers Association (TFA) and is still a member. He regularly plays guitar with the group. He also collected ideas on how to make life work. He made a list then turned it into this book.